THE
ESSENCE OF
VIBRATIONAL
Healing

Volume 1 Bio-Rhythm

L. LEILA DEONARINE

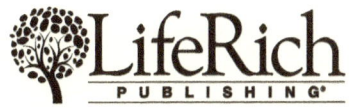

Author photo by Nickayla London Dummet
Interior images by Esther Nicola London

LifeRich Publishing is a registered trademark of The Reader's Digest Association, Inc.

LifeRich Publishing books may be ordered through booksellers or by contacting:

LifeRich Publishing
1663 Liberty Drive
Bloomington, IN 47403
www.liferichpublishing.com
1 (888) 238-8637

Because of the dynamic nature of the Internet, any web addresses or links contained in this book may have changed since publication and may no longer be valid. The views expressed in this work are solely those of the author and do not necessarily reflect the views of the publisher, and the publisher hereby disclaims any responsibility for them.

Any people depicted in stock imagery provided by Thinkstock are models, and such images are being used for illustrative purposes only.
Certain stock imagery © Thinkstock.

ISBN: 978-1-4897-1100-7 (sc)
ISBN: 978-1-4897-1101-4 (e)

Print information available on the last page.

LifeRich Publishing rev. date: 09/14/2017

Contents

Foreword..vii

Acknowledgements xi

Introduction...xiii

Advisory.. xvii

Exercise 1 – Overlapping Palms 1

Exercise 2 – Fingers on the Shoulders............................ 6

Exercise 3 – 1st Thoracic Vertebra.................................. 11

Exercise 4 – Cervical Vertebrae or Neck Bones 16

Exercise 5 – Ears, Pons and Medulla 21

Exercise 6 – Above the Ear.. 26

Exercise 7 – Centre of the Head 31

Exercise 8 – Top of the Head and Forehead...................... 36

Exercise 9 – The Face 41

Exercise 10 – Closure.. 46

Self-Reflection 51

Foreword

This book came about in an early morning self-meditation session on 23rd August 2013.

I placed my hands together, then found myself doing these exercises. I felt so energized. When I was through, it was as though I was propelled to pick up pen and paper and write down the various exercises and the benefits I experienced.

I did. I now share them with anyone who is willing to participate and enjoy Holistic Bio-Rhythmic Healing Therapies.

"I live in the Abundance of the Universe

And

The Universe of Abundance lives in me".

Leila

Acknowledgements

Thanks to the various persons who participated in my workshops, my clients and well-wishers who supported and encouraged me in this New Era Field of Therapeutic Work.

To my family, siblings, relatives, friends, Reiki and Feng Shui Masters, we were meant to be in this circle.

A special thanks to the many deceased mentors who recognized my natural talents and gifts and led me to the doors to be the I am that I am this day.

I express my earnest gratitude to the Finite and Infinite Intelligence of the Universe.

I Thank you All!

Introduction

What is Essence? (In context with Healing)

Essence is the Value, Sensation and Feelings that are beneficial to the esoteric body. It adds flavour that is positive to the sensations of the Mind, Body and Thoughts. For example, essence in food gives a pleasant savour which excites the taste-buds. When the memory and enjoyment of that pleasurable sensation lives on there is a desire to have more and more. That's how I felt with the exercises.

What is healing?

Healing is to make ourselves wholistic, that is to let the physical, social, financial, intellectual, emotional, mental, communicative and spiritual selves within us integrate and resonate as one being.

What is Vibration?

Vibration is rhythmic wave lengths. Our breath has a rhythm, as in the lashing of the waves against land or on the beach. Waterfalls, clocks and music have rhythms or vibrations. The rhythmic pulsating sensations you feel throughout your body, for example, the wrist, forehead, feet, hands and chest are also nerve endings that are sending messages to the brain.

What is your Bio-Rhythm?

Body Rhythm is about 60 to 100 beats per minute. Its variation depends on different factors, such as your age, your emotional stability, your mental thoughts in the moment and your varying health patterns.

Your thoughts

Are

Your vibrations:

Good thoughts

Bring

Good results;

Bad

Unpleasant thoughts

Bring negative

Harmful results,

Circumstances

And

Consequences.

Healing of the body is through the Thought Process of the Mind.

"My Body Heals Through My Mind
My Mind Heals My Body."

Advisory

These Bio-Rhythm exercises are aimed towards Self-Healing, therefore, be advised to continue your visits to your medical practitioner and take your prescribed medication.

These Bio-Rhythm exercises are complementary to achieving better health and assist to maintain a more balanced mind and body.

These are some benefits of the various Vibrational Bio-Rhythm exercises

1. Calms the mind.
2. Relaxes the body.
3. Clears the respiratory tract.
4. Increases oxygen flow to the cells.
5. Awareness of the sensory organs and their functions.
6. Awareness of feeling the rhythm of your body.
7. Releases stress.
8. Balances the physical body structure.
9. Assists in emotional and mental well-being.
10. Relieves insomnia or sleeplessness.
11. Better mobility and control of the motor system.
12. Increases awareness of the pressure points in the body.
13. Increases energy flow.
14. Long–term health benefits with positive thoughts towards self-healing.
15. Releases toxins.

Some persons may experience a change in body temperature, frequency in urinating, diarrhea, constipation, nausea, headache, or even sweating can increase.

Should conditions persist for a period of twenty four to forty eight hours (1 to 2 days), please consult your medical practitioner. Consume well-balanced and regular meals daily.

You are encouraged to keep a journal on each of the various exercises. Every time you practice these Vibrational Bio-Rhythm exercises you may experience different or similar sensations which can be compared on a regular basis.

Each exercise can be done for three (3) minutes. If you feel the need to spend more time on any particular area of the body please do.

Allow yourself to smile while doing these exercises; a relaxing facial expression can help to reset your nervous system.

Exercise 1

Overlapping Palms

Overlap the hand with one palm above the other in an opposite direction, the middle fingers straight over each other and the tips resting lightly on the centre of the palms.

Concentrate on the pulse-beat, vibration or rhythm you may feel from the tips of the fingers and the middle of the palms.

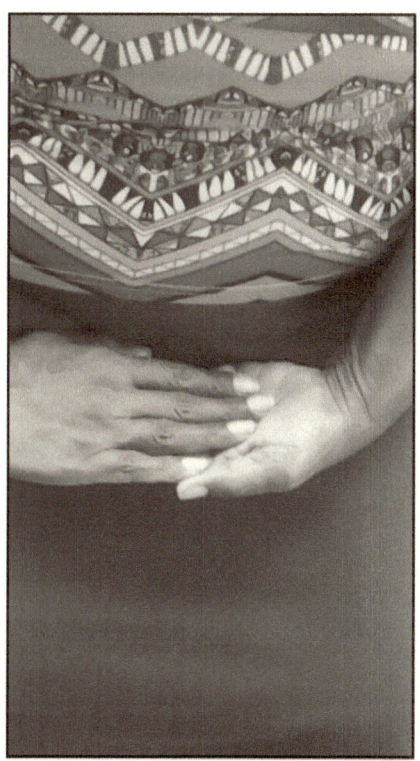

Exercise 1
Overlapping Palms

Exercise 1

Observe the sensations you may experience throughout your body.

- Notice your breathing pattern; is there any change?
- Pay close attention to your feelings at this time.
- Relax the body by allowing your thoughts to flow, try not to concentrate on any particular thought during this time.
- Enjoy the sensations of the pulse-beat throughout your body.

You can record on the journal page after each of the exercises. Every time you do these exercises there may be different or similar sensations and a comparison can be made at a later period.

Exercise 1

Self-evaluate and journal your daily sensations here.

Day1_____

_____

_____

Day2_____

_____

_____

Day3_____

_____

_____

Day4_____

_____

_____

Day5_____

_____

_____

Day6_____

_____

_____

Day7_____

_____

_____

Exercise 2

Fingers on the Shoulders

With palms facing towards the front of the neck, place the tips of the middle and index fingers, with a slight pressure into the soft tissues on the hollow area between the neck and the collar bone.

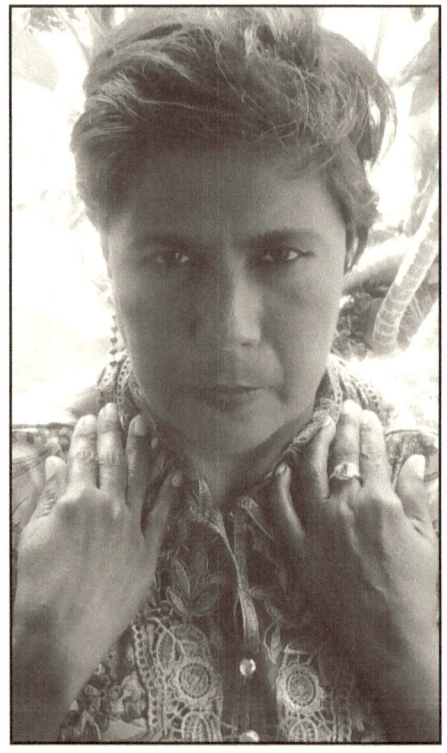

Exercise 2
Fingers on the Shoulders

Exercise 2

Some benefits derived from this exercise should help you to

- Concentrate on your breathing pattern.
- Become more aware of the rhythm of your heart beat.
- Clear the nasal passages.
- Be more alert of the sensations of the inner ear.

Exercise 2

Self-evaluate and journal your daily sensations here.

Day1_____

_____

_____

Day2_____

_____

_____

Day3_____

_____

_____

Day4_____

_____

_____

Day5_____

_____

_____

Day6_____

_____

_____

Day7_____

_____

_____

Exercise 3

1st Thoracic Vertebra

To find the first thoracic vertebra, place your palms across the shoulders then swing your neck slowly from left to right, side to side or front to back.. Slide the palms slightly upward over the back of the neck; letting the middle fingers press very lightly on the middle of the first stationary bone for three minutes.

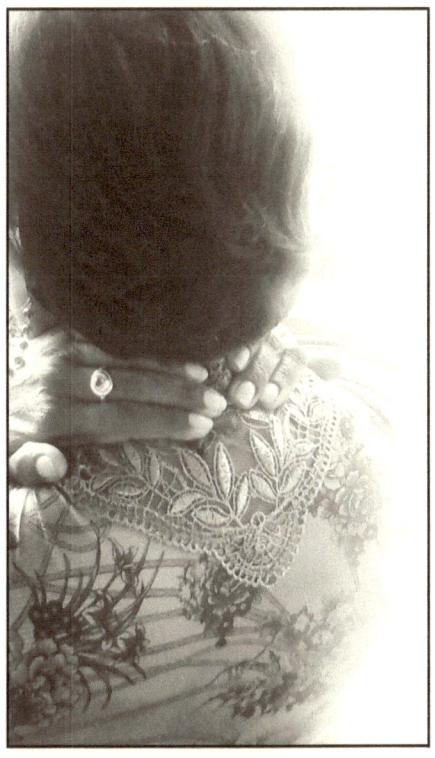

Exercise 3
1st Thoracic Vertebra

Exercise 3

Concentrate and observe the sensation along the spine.

- A more rhythmic pattern of breathing would have been established at this point.
- Notice the areas of the body where you may feel painful sensations.

  Pain can be healthy because it brings an awareness which is an indicator that there is abnormal functioning of a part of the body or its energy centers.

Notify your medical doctor, as soon as possible, of the painful areas along the spine or any other part of the body.

Please be cognizant of your discoveries, make a note of them in your journal for further reference at a later date and time when you are dealing with your self-reflection and evaluation of the various exercises.

Exercise 3

Self-evaluate and journal your daily sensations here.

Day1_____

_____

_____

Day2_____

_____

_____

Day3_____

_____

_____

Day4_____

_____

_____

Day5_____

_____

_____

Day6_____

_____

_____

Day7_____

_____

_____

Exercise 4

Cervical Vertebrae or Neck Bones

Slowly slide palms upwards, under the earlobes, allowing the middle fingers to touch each other and the rest of the fingers closed in, in a relaxed position around the neck for three minutes or more.

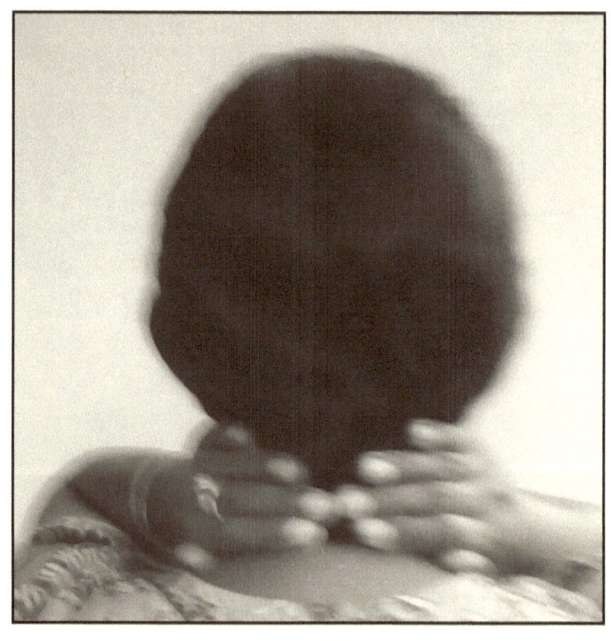

Exercise 4
Cervical Vertebrae or Neck Bones

Exercise 4

Some observations that you should pay attention to

- Notice the feeling of relaxation.
- Do you sense stressful areas across the shoulder or the upper part of the body?

This exercise is a stress-buster. It can be done several times during your waking hours and anywhere during brief moments.

Exercise 4

Self-evaluate and journal your daily sensations here.

Day1_____

_____

_____

Day2_____

_____

_____

Day3_____

_____

_____

Day4_____

_____

_____

Day5_____

_____

_____

Day6_____

_____

_____

Day7_____

_____

_____

Exercise 5

Ears, Pons and Medulla

Place the middle of the palm very lightly on each ear which would be completely covered. The tips of the middle fingers should be resting on the hollow area at the centre above the cervical vertebrae.

Should there be difficulty in breathing, slowly breathe in through the nostrils and breathe out through the lips. Perhaps the palms are placed too tightly over the ears; so, gently ease the pressure of the palms.

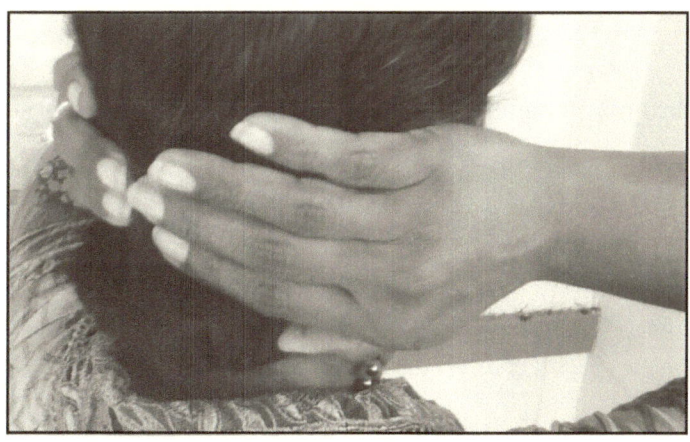

Exercise 5
Ears, Pons and Medulla

Exercise 5

Some benefits you may experience.

- It helps to clear the nasal passages.
- Increases rhythmic breathing.
- Increases blood flow.
- Relaxes the body.
- Relieves insomnia/sleeplessness.
- Calms the nervous system.
- Increases concentration.

This is an excellent exercise for children and stressful situations.

Journal in details the sensation you encounter in this exercise.

There are many benefits in this one and it can be done anywhere, for example, dealing with a stressful situation, at home, work, before sleep or after waking up, travelling as a passenger, walking or just relaxing.

Exercise 5

Self-evaluate and journal your daily sensations here.

Day1_____
_____
_____

Day2_____
_____
_____

Day3_____
_____
_____

Day4_____
_____
_____

Day5_____
_____
_____

Day6_____
_____
_____

Day7_____
_____
_____

Exercise 6

Above the Ear

Slide hands above the ears letting the tips of the middle fingers touch each other allowing the essence of the bio-rhythm vibrations to serenade the pituitary gland.

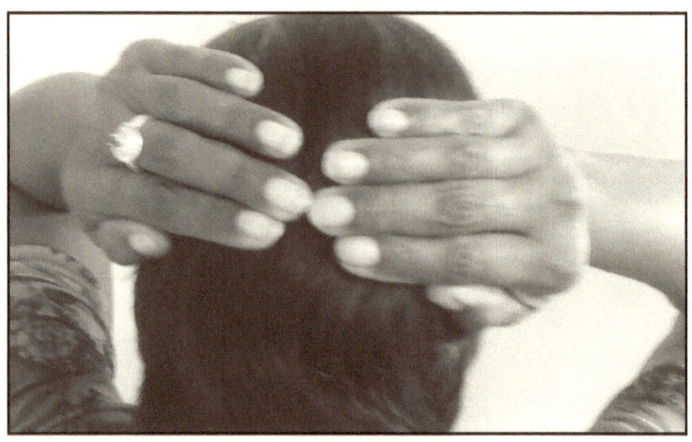

Exercise 6
Above the Ears

Exercise 6

Some benefits derived

- More efficient function of the pituitary gland.
- Increases awareness on the sensory organs.
- Increases flow of the blood.
- Helps with digestion.

Exercise 6

Self-evaluate and journal your daily sensations here.

Day1_____

_____

_____

Day2_____

_____

_____

Day3_____

_____

_____

Day4_____

_____

_____

Day5_____

_____

_____

Day6_____

_____

_____

Day7_____

_____

_____

Exercise 7

Centre of the Head

Pivot the palms across the centre of the head with the tips of the middle fingers touching each other; sensing the vibrations on the pineal gland.

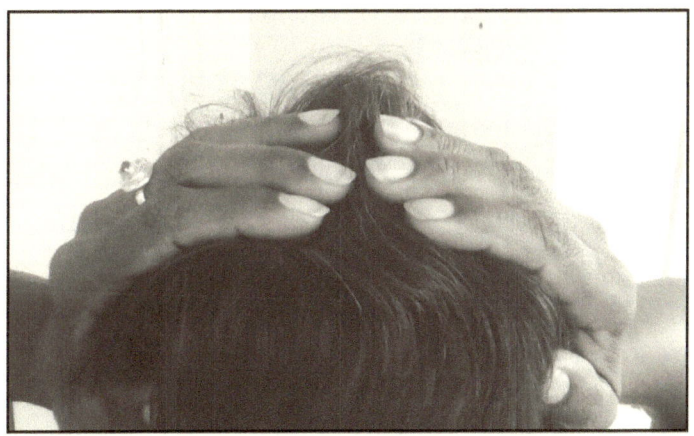

Exercise 7
Centre of the Head

Exercise 7

This exercise vibrates on the pineal gland

Some benefits you may experience

- More efficient function on the pineal gland.
- Releases toxin.
- Increases energy flow.
- Having better mobility and control of the motor system.
- Helps to build clarity in thinking.
- Improves awareness.

Journal every sensation so that a comparison can be made of what it felt like on the first day when this exercise was done to what it was on the fifth day or the ninth day or the following months.

Record your progress, so that you can share your knowledge with someone and give back to the Universe.

Exercise 7

Self-evaluate and journal your daily sensations here.

Day1_____

_____

_____

Day2_____

_____

_____

Day3_____

_____

_____

Day4_____

_____

_____

Day5_____

_____

_____

Day6_____

_____

_____

Day7_____

_____

_____

Exercise 8

Top of the Head and Forehead

Shift the hands from the centre to the top of the head, the tips of the middle fingers touching each other. You may wish to keep the hands a little longer on this area, please do.

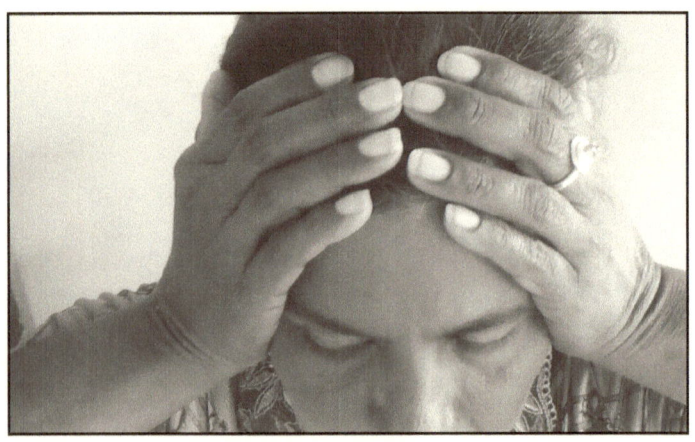

Exercise 8
Top of the Head and Forehead

Exercise 8

Some benefits you may notice

- Increase function of the immunity system
- Release and relieve, physical, mental, and emotional stress.
- Relax the mind, body and spirit.
- Clear the respiratory tract.
- Balance the body's stature.
- Release toxic energy
- Assist in healing the mind, body and spirit.
- Increase energy levels.

Record your personal benefits in details.

Exercise 8

Self-evaluate and journal your daily sensations here.

Day1_____

_____

_____

Day2_____

_____

_____

Day3_____

_____

_____

Day4_____

_____

_____

Day5_____

_____

_____

Day6_____

_____

_____

Day7_____

_____

_____

Exercise 9

The Face

Spread the fingers and palms across the face. The fifth or smallest fingers are at the centre of the brows which is at the beginning of the nose bridge. The index fingers are on either side of the forehead and the thumbs are below the ear.

Sense the vibrations and internalized them with positive thoughts of healing, joy, laughter, humour and prosperity of the body, mind and spirit.

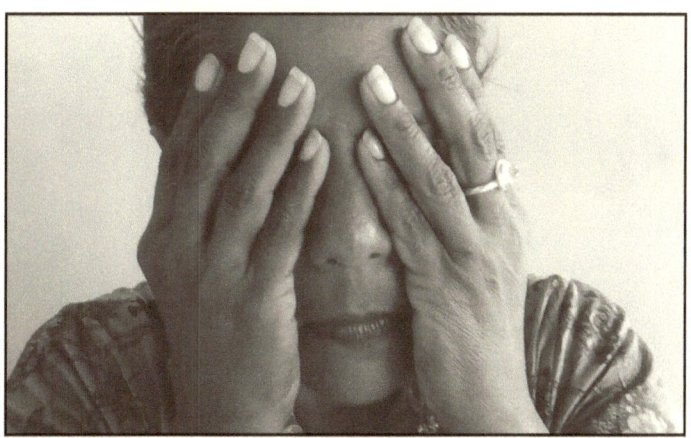

Exercise 9
The Face

Exercise 9

Enjoy the sensations of the Vibrational Bio-Rhythm on the face which can

- Balance the energy flow of the body.
- Increase blood circulation.
- Increase awareness of the bodily functions of each organ, especially the skin.
- Improve immunity.
- Sense feelings of relaxation.
- Increase sensations of the five senses
- Help the digestive system.

Exercise 9

Self-evaluate and journal your daily sensations here.

Day1_____

_____

_____

Day2_____

_____

_____

Day3_____

_____

_____

Day4_____

_____

_____

Day5_____

_____

_____

Day6_____

_____

_____

Day7_____

_____

_____

Exercise 10

Closure

Attitude of Gratitude

With this procedure of Vibrational Pulse on the body, you are now ending with an Attitude of Gratitude.

Place one hand slightly cupped with the palm under the collar-bone and the other across the chest.

Let go and surrender to the pulsating rhythms throughout your body.

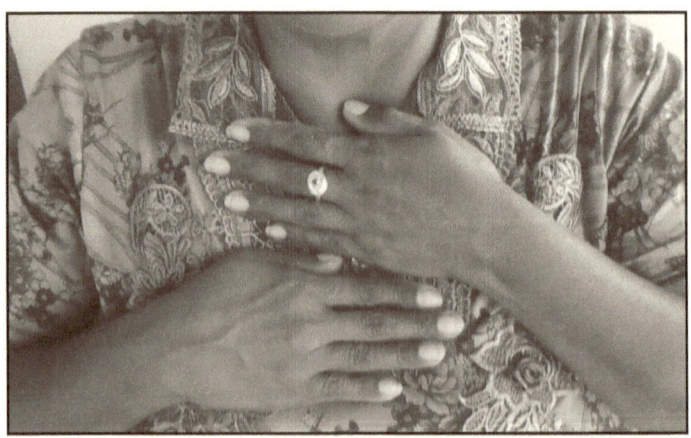

Exercise 10
Closure

Exercise 10

This is your MOMENT of GRATITUDE.

Allow yourself to flow in thought, giving thanks in the Spirit of Gratitude.

You can say to yourself,

"My body is now relaxed, I am or I feel comfortable with myself and the various sensations that were aroused to bring to me further awareness of my being. Thank you, for I live in the abundant blessings of the UNIVERSE."

Notice I have not written any benefits, observations or sensations here.

From the feedback I received in the various workshops that I had done, many persons mentioned that they were overcome with deep self-awareness and emotional expression of gratitude towards their bodies.

You can email me at leila-theessenceofvibrationalhealing06@outlook.com and express your Attitude of Gratitude.

Exercise 10

Self-evaluate and journal your daily sensations here.

Day1_____

_____

_____

Day2_____

_____

_____

Day3_____

_____

_____

Day4_____

_____

_____

Day5_____

_____

_____

Day6_____

_____

_____

Day7_____

_____

_____

Self-Reflection

You have done those exercises at least once for the day, what changes have you noticed to your body over the past seven (7) days or weeks?

For example, on

Day1, Week1
I felt relaxed, less stressful at work, my back pain decreased and my breathing was less troublesome. The exercises helped to clear my sinus and respiratory tract. I was able to cope with a mild migraine headache after exercise 5.

Day5 Week2
I was a more relaxed person. I was becoming more aware of my breath and breathing. My facial muscles were so relaxed that my natural smile was more noticeable. I had become more aware of my physical self; my mind was more alert and appreciative of my environment.

Day 7 Week 3
It felt great as though my physical body was resonating in one accord with mind and spirit being. My emotional self was in more control over the physical self and I experience acute clarity mentally. Most of the internal pains are no longer there. I can concentrate more easily on the various things I have to do daily.

Daily Self-Reflection of the 1st week

Day1_____

_____

_____

Day2_____

_____

_____

Day3_____

_____

_____

Day4_____

_____

_____

Day5_____

_____

_____

Day6_____

_____

_____

Day7_____

_____

_____

Daily Self-Reflection of the 2nd week

Day1_____

_____

_____

Day2_____

_____

_____

Day3_____

_____

_____

Day4_____

_____

_____

Day5_____

_____

_____

Day6_____

_____

_____

Day7_____

_____

_____

Daily Self-Reflection of the 3rd week

Day1_____

_____

_____

Day2_____

_____

_____

Day3_____

_____

_____

Day4_____

_____

_____

Day5_____

_____

_____

Day6_____

_____

_____

Day7_____

_____

_____

www.ingramcontent.com/pod-product-compliance
Lightning Source LLC
Chambersburg PA
CBHW050429290526
45786CB00003B/1455